THE RESILIENT WARRIOR

Jerry Yellin

Dr. Sarina Grosswald

TotalRecall Publications
1103 Middlecreek
Friendswood, TX 77536

To Warriors of all Wars

RESILIENCE

"The ability to recover
from or adjust easily to
misfortune or change."

Webster's Dictionary

Jerry Yellin

Jerry Yellin was a P-51 pilot in WWII who flew nineteen missions over Japan. Jerry and his wife of sixty-one years, Helene, have four sons and six grandchildren—three living in America and three in Japan. Jerry is a member of the Military Writers Society of America; author of three award-winning books, *Of War and Weddings*, *The Blackened Canteen*, and *The Letter*; and an honorary board member of the Iwo Jima Association of America.

http://www.JerryYellin.com
jerry@lisco.com

Dr. Sarina J. Grosswald

Dr. Sarina J. Grosswald, an expert in cognitive learning, is Director of Research for Operation Warrior Wellness of the David Lynch Foundation. She has been a principal on research teams studying the effects of meditation on stress-related disorders, including Post-Traumatic Stress Disorder (PTSD) in veterans of the Iraq and Afghanistan wars. Her first-of-its-kind research on the effects of the Transcendental Meditation program on children with ADHD has received worldwide media attention. Dr. Grosswald has published and lectured widely in the fields of medicine and education. In addition to scholarly journals, her work has been featured in *US News and World Report*, *Business Week*, *Newsweek*, *International Herald Tribune*, *Barron's*, *ABC News*, and *PBS*.

Books by award-winning Military Writers Society of America author Jerry Yellin

The Blackened Canteen

ISBN-13: 9781421890180

"On June 20, 1945, just before the end of the war, 123 American bombers took off from the island of Guam for an attack on Shizuoka, a Japanese city at the foot of Mount Fuji. The raid destroyed two-thirds of the city, taking the lives of two thousand of its citizens and twenty-three American airmen."

Of War and Weddings

ISBN-13: 9780963850256

"*Of War and Weddings* is a moving and compelling true story of bitter wartime enemies who find peace through their children's marriage. A mysterious force that weaves its way into the lives of the Yellin and Yamakawa families ends up healing the wounds of war and nurturing a legacy of freedom and understanding for the children of America and Japan."

The Letter

ISBN-13: 9781590957332

"*The Letter* is a story about a powerful United States Senator, raised as a Fundamental Christian, who finds out his parents were a Catholic woman and a Jewish father when he reads a letter sent by his dying birth mother to his birth father. The suspense, twists and turns are unique. A must read!"

Learning to meditate

is the greatest gift

you can give yourself in
this life.

For it is only through
meditation

That you can undertake
the journey

To discover your true
nature,

And so find the stability
and confidence

You will need to live and
die well.

Sogyal Rinpoche

Acknowledgment

This book is a direct outcome of the noble work of the award-winning filmmaker David Lynch and the David Lynch Foundation. David learned the Transcendental Meditation® technique in 1973 and established his Foundation in 2005 to ensure that anyone suffering from traumatic stress who wants to learn to meditate can do so. In the past five years the David Lynch Foundation has provided scholarships for more than 150,000 people—including veterans and students—to learn the TM® technique and thereby reduce stress, improve health and creativity, and promote inner peace.

After the tragic suicide of a close friend's son, a young man named Dory Klock who served eight years in the Army, I approached my dear friend Bob Roth, who is executive director of the David Lynch Foundation. I asked him about the possibility of creating a Veterans Division of the Foundation to raise funds to teach the TM technique to returning warriors suffering from post-traumatic stress disorder. Bob's immediate and resounding response was: "YES—and you will have the support of the entire Foundation." So my deepest and heartfelt thanks go to those in the David Lynch Foundation, including Bob, David Lynch, Dr. John Hagelin, Julia and Chris Busch, and all the others who work so diligently behind the scenes. Thank you.

Without the knowledge and help of my colleague, Dr. Sarina Grosswald, a renowned researcher on the effects of TM practice on stress, health, and cognitive learning, this book would not have been completed, much less worthwhile. Colonel Brian Rees, M.D., a veteran of four tours in Afghanistan and Iraq, has made several key suggestions and edits of the manuscript, even while performing his military duties overseas. Ed Schloeman, a Marine Vietnam veteran whom I met on Iwo Jima in March 2010, has been a true supporter and has shared my goals since day one.

Bruce Moran of Total Recall Press has enthusiastically supported this project in every way. I am grateful for his support and friendship, and for our business relationship.

As always, writing and fundraising take time. Time away from Helene, my wife of sixty-one years, is difficult for both of us. But she too recognizes the importance of this project, and her support of my activities is especially important. She gives her support at times hesitantly—because she feels (not unreasonably!) that at my age of 86 years I am too old to do what I do—but she always gives it with love and enthusiasm.

Prologue

It has been said that the only warriors who do not suffer after being in combat are those who were killed. I cannot attest to that for all battle-tested warriors, but I certainly can for one — me.

Some years ago, a 13-year-old eighth-grade student from the Fairfield Middle School in Fairfield, Iowa, asked me, "Were you wounded in the war?"

For many years, I had been invited to Mrs. Broz's class to talk about my wartime experiences. Though I had been asked and had answered many questions, this one was different. I paused, thought deeply, and replied.

"Yes, I was wounded, seriously wounded, but it was not a wound that anyone could see and fix." The question gave me pause to think about warriors of all the wars, whose wounds, like mine, were unseen, untreated, and debilitating, even though no blood was shed.

I spent a sleepless night wondering if my answer had satisfied him...or me. What was there about my military service that left me so hopeless and so helpless when I returned home to civilian life? Was it me? The military? The combat?

In order to understand what happened to me, and to many others who serve their country in war, I must tell you about our experiences. When we are sent to war, we do not question why: Those questions are matters for others. The reality of war, however, and the damage it does both physically and mentally, is real, long-lasting, devastating, and costly. And it affects not just those who fight but also all who love them—friends and family.

In this book I tell my story and the story of others. My hope is that what I describe, including the relief we've found, will help others who have served and endured, and— like me—quietly suffered, to finally find what could lift the weight from our shoulders and allow us to enjoy life again.

Table of Contents

Chapter 1:
My War

I was seventeen on December 7, 1941, the day the Japanese attacked Pearl Harbor. It felt as if someone had invaded my home, and I had to do something about it. Two months later— on my eighteenth birthday, February 15, 1942—I enlisted in the Army Air Corps as an Aviation Cadet in waiting. In August 1942, after taking all of the examinations, physical and mental, I was inducted into the Army Air Corps. My training took me to Nashville, Santa Ana, Thunderbird Field in Phoenix, Marana Army Air Base in Tucson, and Luke Field in Phoenix, where I graduated as a fighter pilot in August 1943. I joined the 78th Fighter Squadron on Oahu in October 1943.

I quickly became familiar with death. In December, Bill Sutherland, the CO of the 78th, was killed in a midair collision with Howard Edmondson. Edmondson was killed a few months later when he flew his plane into the sea. Ed Green lost his life when he couldn't pull his P-47 out of a flat spin, and both Bob Ferris and John Lindner died when their P-51's exploded over Bellows Field. I attended services for all five of my friends and squadron mates. I mourned their losses but never thought it could happen to me.

On March 7, 1945, our squadron landed on Iwo Jima, on a dirt runway at the foot of Mount Suribachi. I looked out at the landscape as I taxied my P-51 Mustang to our parking area, and saw huge piles of dead Japanese soldiers being pushed into mass graves. The sight and smell is indelibly imprinted on my mind. It was a shocking sight for a young man to see as he entered his 21st year.

The fighting had been fierce on this eight-square-mile island, 650 miles from Japan.

Twenty-one thousand Japanese soldiers lost their lives there. Our squadron area was next to a Marine mortuary where hundreds of dead Marines were being readied for burial, a ritual that continued until the remains of nearly 7,000 American Marines were buried in the cemetery.

I flew nineteen long-range missions over Japan from Iwo Jima, flying with eleven other young pilots, all of them friends, who did not return home.

Fred White bailed out of his P-51 on April 12, 1945, and his parachute did not open. Lee Barghaer lost his life when the Japanese exploded a device under his plane as he strafed the runway at Chichi Jima. Dick Schroeppel was hit when he was following me on a strafing run on the airfield of that small island 100 miles from our base on Iwo. He bailed out, ran to the coastline, swam out to sea and climbed into a large lifeboat that was dropped by a B-17. Mortar fire got him and the boat was sunk by rockets with his body in it.

On May 30th, 1945, I shot down a Zero over Tokyo. My wingman, Danny Mathis, also hit the Japanese plane, and we were each credited with half a kill.

I had a toothache when we landed back at Iwo. I ended up having my four wisdom teeth pulled, and I was grounded. Danny was assigned my plane, Dorrie R, and my spot for an escort mission over Osaka on June 1. The squadron took off early in the morning. An hour after takeoff they were led into a huge weather front by the navigating B-29. In the clouds a few pilots spun out and knocked twenty-seven fighter planes out of the sky like bowling pins. Twenty-five pilots were killed, including Danny in my plane, and Jack Nelson from the 78th.

Jack Wrightman crash landed his P-51 in Japan, was captured and died of a broken back in Kempai Tai, a Japanese prisoner-of-war camp. His classmates, Wightman and Wayland, also died in combat over Japan.

On July 8, 1945, Al Sherren, my classmate

from flying school, called in, "I'm hit and can't see," and he was gone. Robert "Pudgy" Carr also disappeared on that day. He was my tent mate.

I learned about the bombing of Hiroshima when I returned from an eight-hour mission on August 6, 1945. Phil Maher jumped on my wing and shouted, "It's over, one bomb, one city, and it's over." I thought he was crazy but it was true. Hiroshima was gone. No more guys getting killed, no more butt-breaking eight-hour missions. And our motto "Back Alive in '45" would come true.

But it wasn't to be. On August 13th a mission statement was posted on the bulletin board: Take off tomorrow, August 14 at 0700, for a fighter sweep of airfields near Tokyo.

At the afternoon briefing, Jim Tapp, our Commanding Officer and the Squadron leader for the 14th was asked, "How come another mission, sir?"

"We have to keep them honest," Tapp replied. "We know the war is almost over.

Preparations have been made to abort should that happen during the flight up or on the mission itself, and it probably will. B-17's and Navy destroyers will be in place to broadcast the codeword 'Ohio' on the entire route to Japan. When we hear it we'll do a 180 and return to Hotrocks"—the code word for Iwo Jima.

Phil Schlamberg, 19 years old from Brooklyn, was assigned to my wing in Blue flight. He leaned over to me during the briefing and whispered, "If I go, Captain, I won't come back." Startled, I asked, "Why?" "Just a feeling," he replied.

After the briefing, I told Tapp what Phil had said. "I don't have a replacement for him, Jerry," Tapp told me. "Only Doc Lewis can get him off the mission, but Schlamberg will have to agree to see him."

"No way. No way will I see Doc," Phil said, quite emphatically.

Just before takeoff the next morning I told Phil, "Just stick close on my wing. Don't even think of moving away from a tight position. We'll be okay. It will be over before we reach the target."

No one heard the codeword "Ohio" on the flight to Japan, or when we reached the coast and had to drop our external wing tanks. We dropped our tanks, found our targets, and strafed the airfields. We needed ninety gallons of fuel to return to Iwo from Japan. When someone called, "Ninety gallons," we formed up, and headed out to sea and to our navigating B-29. Phil was tucked in close on my wing. I looked over, gave him a "thumbs up," and led the flight into some clouds. When we came through the clouds Phil was gone. No radio contact, no visual sighting, just gone.

When we landed on Iwo we found out that the war had been over for three hours, while we were still fighting. Phil Schlamberg must have been the last man killed on a combat mission over Japan in World War II. He didn't have to die.

Chapter 2:
Discharged

I returned home to New Jersey in December 1945. I reported to Fort Monmouth in Eatontown, New Jersey, where I was given a physical, handed my discharge papers, and sent home to Hillside. I was a former Captain, combat squadron leader, and fighter pilot. But now, emotionally I was just a 17-year-old high school graduate. I was a lost soul, with no one to talk to and no real life experiences to fall back on.

Just after Christmas, I drove to Brooklyn, New York, to meet Phil Schlamberg's family and to bring them Phil's wings and Lieutenant's bars. Phil's mother didn't want to meet me, but his sisters did. I gave them his possessions, told them what a wonderful guy he was and how he died. It was heartbreaking for them and difficult for me, very difficult.

When I was saying goodbye, his mother looked at me and said, "It should have been you who was killed, Captain, not my son Phillip. I hope you never sleep another night in your life, like I can't."

I sat on their front stoop as the snow collected at my feet for an hour before I could get up and leave their house.

For two years I had been a valued member of a large team with only one purpose—to win the war. Four hundred men, working their specialty—armorers, radiomen, crew chiefs, parachute riggers—all with one goal, keeping 30 to 35 airplanes in perfect flying condition so we fighter pilots could take them into combat. Every day we knew what we were doing and why. The pilots were the stars, the chosen few. The missions were long; the highs were higher than anything anyone could imagine. The camaraderie, our purity of purpose, even the danger never clouded our vision.

I had been living with warriors for a long time. We ate together, played together, trained together, and, for a few of us, flew together. Our days in training were long and fruitful.

Our goal as a squadron was to build confidence in our abilities, learn the complexities of our airplane, and become a working unit that would hold up in combat with our enemy.

Individual mentality became team mentality. Single-engine fighter pilots had a lot of freedom when they flew their high-performance airplanes. But that freedom of thought and action had to be molded into a functioning unit if we were to be successful. Hours of formation flying, doing sixteen-plane aerobatics, loops, and slow rolls, made us comfortable with each other. It was a learning experience like none other.

I learned a lot about myself. My abilities to fly an airplane grew exponentially with every hour in the sky. In time I became an element leader, a leader of a two-man flight that was half of a four-man team working the sky together as part of a sixteen-airplane squadron.

We were highly trained fighter pilots looking for action every time we left for a mission over Japan.

That the 78th Fighter Squadron, my squadron for two years—the only squadron I ever flew with—was the best, was unquestionable. Then in one minute it was over. The war ended; our reason for living was gone.

Life for me from 1946 to 1975 was empty. The highs I had experienced in combat became the lows of daily living. I had absolutely no connection to my parents, my sister, my relatives, or my friends. I listened to some of the guys I knew talk about their experiences in combat, and I knew they had never been in a battle, let alone a war zone. No one I knew who had seen their friends die could talk about it. I wasn't interested in going to college, even though it was free with the G.I. Bill. The Army Air Corps had trained me and prepared me to fly combat missions, but there was no training on how to fit into society when the war was over and I stopped flying.

I met my future wife, Helene, on Good Friday in 1949. We were engaged on Memorial Day, and married on October 22. Her parents furnished an apartment for us in West Orange, New Jersey. I commuted to New York where I worked for her father, and hated every day. My escape was golf, an escape I desperately needed. Our first son was born in November 1950 and our fourth was born in August 1960. But I couldn't find contentment, any reason to succeed, any connection to anyone that had meaning or value. I was depressed, unhappy, and lonely even though surrounded by my family.

That feeling of disconnect, lack of emotions, restlessness, and the empty feeling of hopelessness lasted until 1975. I heard words that described my condition as "battle fatigue" or "shell shocked." Now that condition is known as "post-traumatic stress disorder (PTSD)." Every soldier who has been in combat lives with his memories, and suffers silently.

One afternoon in 1975, Helene was watching the *Merv Griffin Show* on television. Merv's guest that day was Maharishi Mahesh Yogi, a teacher from India who brought Transcendental Meditation®, an ancient form of meditation, from India to the United States. Helene was fascinated and wanted to learn more. Her search led her to a Transcendental Meditation Center in North Miami Beach, Florida. Excited, she expressed her desire to learn TM to our second son, Steven, who had just graduated from the University of Pennsylvania. Steven was on the Penn tennis team, and the team was leaving for a series of matches in England, so he asked Helene to wait to learn to meditate until he came back in late June.

Both Helene and Steven learned Transcendental Meditation in August 1975, and I learned one month later. It was the beginning of a huge metamorphosis in my life. After a few weeks of twice-a-day meditations, my attitude toward myself began to change. I felt a connection to my inner self. My anger and restlessness began to dissipate, and a calmness that I never knew before became apparent, not only to me but to my family as well. As time progressed I found myself thinking differently about the world around me, and found a direction that had been missing in my life. I welcomed the change eagerly, and TM became part of my routine every morning and every evening. I have been doing it now for thirty-five years. It saved my life.

Chapter 3:
Civilian Life, 1945-2010

But what about my family—and the families of others who suffer from PTSD? I had a sister six years younger than me, a father and mother who loved me, and my wife's parents who loved her and took me to be their daughter's perfect husband. Did they suffer because of my PTSD?

It wasn't apparent to me then, but it is now. My behavior was off the wall for the first twenty-six years of my marriage. Too many jobs, too many moves, too much golf. I can't imagine what they were thinking, and at the time I really didn't care. It wasn't until years later that I was able to care about the people I loved in the same way I had before I went to war.

I played a lot of golf with Jerry Pisano before he turned pro. One day we were on the tenth hole at Old Orchard, and he looked at me and said, "Jerry, you play golf for the wrong reason." I didn't know what he was talking about. Didn't everyone play golf like it was combat: to win, to beat the golf course and your opponents?

I had some friends who did business with my father-in-law's company. The family often contacted my friends, to have them intercede and try to find out what was going on in my head. When asked, I had no answers. I didn't really know that I was a problem, or was causing problems for others.

When we moved far away, really far away, my wife's parents pleaded for her to get a divorce: to come home, live near them, come back, live near her family again. She was torn between her love and loyalty to me and our children, and her connection to her parents. They offered her money—whatever she wanted or needed. Her refusal and her devotion to me caused her a lot of anxious days and nights. It created a breach in her relationship with her parents. In their eyes, I was the cause of those problems. And I was, but I didn't know it then. Only now, so many years later, do I recognize the damage I had done to really good people.

Is the same thing happening today? Of course, and in large numbers, by those who have returned as broken as I had been. Families are broken apart every day by the out-of-control behavior of decent, caring, loving young men and women who went to war. They are coming home as strangers. They speak a different language, and see life through the eyes of a warrior trained to kill, not to live life as a civilian.

In early 2010, I was introduced to a young man, Dory Klock, an eight-year Army veteran who fought in Bosnia. He was having difficulty adjusting and keeping a job, and was fighting drugs and alcohol. I knew his inner struggles all too well. His wife and two daughters were suffering with him. His mom, my friend Lin, was beside herself. Then one day Lin called and asked me if I could help her out.

"Sure, Lin, anything," I told her.

She began weeping; she couldn't speak. Finally she asked, "Can you help me put Dory's medals and ribbons on his dress uniform? We want to bury him in it, Jerry. He committed suicide yesterday."

Lin brought Dory's uniform to my home, and I put the medals and insignias in place. When Lin left, I broke down. My thoughts ran wild with the suffering so many are experiencing from the life and death of soldiers and marines who go into combat and have nothing to hold on to when they come home. The training might teach them about the highs experienced in combat, but there is no training for the experiences of normal life when the fighting is over.

Now in 2011, our country is finally recognizing the tremendous stress and pressure put on soldiers and families from the two wars we have been fighting in Iraq and Afghanistan.

How is it possible that we civilians, who

served our country then and now, are expected to learn to fight and kill, to be at war one day, and then enter life again as if nothing had happened? How could the military leaders of my day expect a warrior to return from the horror of Iwo Jima—a battle involving 90,000 soldiers on a small island where 28,000 people died—and just resume leading a normal life?

Can we expect the veterans of the wars in Iraq and Afghanistan to return from their horrors and experiences and integrate back into a normal routine without something deep and meaningful to hold onto? I couldn't. And neither can they. This book will explain why, and offer a time-tested solution as to how we can help our veterans and their families.

There is a poignant scene in the film *Saving Private Ryan*. An elderly, grey-haired man is walking with his family among gravestones in a military cemetery. He stops in front of a grave, bows his head, wipes away a tear, and says to all, "Tell me I am a good man."

Obviously he had been a soldier, and even

after so many years of living in peace, he needed to know that he was an okay guy to his wife and children.

I trained and flew with Leo Evans in Hawaii and on Iwo Jima. Leo was from Butte, Montana. Leo survived the war, found a loving wife, and raised nine children. Today he is in a Veterans Hospital in Montana, with dementia. He didn't recognize his wife before she passed away, nor did he know any of his children. When his son Troy visits him, all Leo talks about is Iwo Jima, his time spent there, and the experiences so deeply etched in his mind.

It is necessary to examine the lives of our young military troops and the lives of their families now, not 20 or 30 or 40 years after they return from battle.

My experience with Lin Klock and her son Dory led me to seek funding to help veterans. I contacted Bob Roth, executive director of the David Lynch Foundation, about opening a Veterans Affairs Division and teaching Transcendental Meditation to veterans suffering from PTSD.

The David Lynch Foundation was originally established to ensure that any young person in America who wanted to learn and practice the Transcendental Meditation program could do so. (To date, the Foundation has provided scholarships for more than 150,000 students to learn to meditate, in the U.S. and around the world.) The TM technique is recognized by doctors and scientists as the most thoroughly researched and widely practiced program in the world for developing the creative potential of the brain and mind, improving health, reducing stress and stress-related disorders, and improving performance.

David Lynch agreed that helping veterans and their families must be a priority, so we launched Operation Warrior Wellness. We added to our team of experts Sarina J. Grosswald, Ed.D., a researcher and expert on TM and stress-related disorders; Ed Schloeman, a retired Marine from the Vietnam war whom I met on Iwo Jima in March 2010;

and Colonel Brian Rees, an active-duty Army surgeon who, at this writing, is serving his fourth tour of duty in Iraq/Afghanistan. Our only purpose is to help our veterans and their families find a vehicle that can help them return to a normal life.

I know from my experiences as an active warrior fighting for my country, and as a returning warrior who suffered from what is now known as post-traumatic stress disorder, that the problem is overwhelming our nation.

I also know that each and every PTSD victim needs a vehicle, a methodology that will help him or her help themselves. Antipsychotic and antidepressant drugs are used extensively, but are extremely costly, especially over the long haul, and do not provide a cure. Many PTSD victims turn to alcohol and recreational drugs as a temporary escape from problems. Many have also taken their lives. I know that mental health professionals provide excellent care, but that care is dependent on complete willingness and cooperation from the patient. And it takes a long, long time. America does not have that time now. We are in crisis.

The best solution for me came when I discovered Transcendental Meditation, a technique that allowed me to reach deep within myself, to find the calm and silence deep within my mind, which gave me the means to eliminate stress and the time to reflect on my role in life as a husband, father, and provider. TM connected me to myself and to the natural world that surrounds us all.

PTSD is a serious illness and a threat to all who surround those afflicted: wives or husbands, parents, children, friends, and family. TM can help everyone help their loved ones and themselves, not for just a month or two, but for life. It is a proven, scientifically researched, non-religious modality, learned once, and then always available to you. Operation Warrior Wellness is ready, willing, and able to make it happen now.

Chapter 4:
Reflection, 2011

I am writing this as an 87-year-old man reflecting on how my military experiences affected my life. In doing so, I have come to the realization that I actually loved the experience of war, more than life itself. I remember my thoughts so vividly after my wingman and friend Danny Mathis was killed. He died in a midair collision while flying my P-51, Dorrie R. I felt a terrible loss— my airplane was gone; I had no weapon.

The way of the warrior, in and of itself, was addictive to me. I am not a scientist; I don't know what happens chemically to the mind while in combat. But I do know I enjoyed flying, fighting, and being part of an incredible team—my squadron, the 78th.

I can only imagine what goes on in the minds of athletes, team players, boxers, tennis players, and golfers when they approach the age when they can no longer compete at their highest level. Many stay too long; many lose their ability to function; many become addicted to something just to hold on to the "high" of competition. The feeling of emptiness is devastating. I faced that empty feeling for many, many years, from the age of 21 to 51. Then I learned Transcendental Meditation.

Those of us who have been to war, those of us who have experienced the highs of combat as warriors, also experience the lows and the emptiness of non-action more profoundly than non-warriors. Many veterans of war find an escape, an addiction like drugs or alcohol or gambling when they return from war. This is evident in the increasing rates of PTSD, suicides, and mental health problems in the military, which are now overwhelming. And it is not only the young men and women who are serving or have served our country who are suffering from the hidden wounds of war. Their immediate and extended family and friends are victims, too. This is not a condition that will go away soon. It will require long-term, expensive care. PTSD requires an approach that can bring some immediate and long-lasting relief. For me, the balance I've felt these past thirty-five years has been realized through my meditation.

As I tried to cope when I got back, my addiction was golf. When I returned from the war at the age of 21, I was lost. I joined a golf club, became the club champion when I was 23, and thought seriously of turning professional, which of course I never did. I would play for six, seven, or eight hours a day, to escape the deep disconnect I felt from everything and everyone around me.

I got married and a year later, November 6, 1950, our first son was born. I had no career, no real ambition. I tried to be a good father and husband. I wanted to remain in one place and send my children to the same school each year. While I was growing up, I went to six different grammar schools in four different cities. We moved every October during the depression years from 1929 through 1940.

I wanted more for my children than I had. But I was deeply flawed from my experiences in the war, and the only place I could do really well and compete at the highest level was on the golf course. So that is what I turned to.

Every evening I hit balls in the back yard. I even had my young sons stationed near their sandbox to catch my shots. I was good, very good. I played a lot, sometimes in tournaments for four days in a row, sometimes once or twice during the week, and always on Saturdays and Sundays, summer and winter. I was not playing for pleasure. I was playing just to escape from who I was and what I dreaded doing every day.

Now I realize my behavior was a real sickness that caused a lot of grief for everyone around me for many years.

Through Transcendental Meditation, I was able to find my balance and remember who I really am. When I close my eyes and meditate, the outer world just disappears from my awareness. Silence surrounds me. Even though I have thoughts, there is a deep, deep calm all around me. The ring of a telephone fades into the background; I continue to feel the peace of my own consciousness. Time has no reference. In fact, when I open my eyes I'm surprised that so much time has passed so quickly.

I enjoy the experience very much, and I know that meditation has connected me in a very personal way to everyone and everything around me. That feeling stays with me throughout the day. I no longer need an escape. I am a better person because of TM.

Chapter 5:
Suffering Soldiers

David George was eighteen when he joined the Army in 2002. His father had served in the Navy. As a young man David attended military school, and dreamed of going to West Point when he graduated from high school. But 9/11 changed all that. As a patriotic duty, he joined the Army. Trained as a 60-MM-mortar man, he shipped out to Baghdad in April 2003, two months after he finished basic training.

Like so many combat veterans, David had a difficult time talking to me about his war and his time in Iraq. He told me that in December 2004, a car ran through the gate of his unit's compound. The guards shot at the car and kept shooting, killing the two men inside. But before the bombers died they detonated a bomb in the car, injuring 50 American soldiers, including David. He recovered from his injuries, but the sight of bodies and of death remained with him.

A few months after the explosion, David returned home to Fort Campbell. One day while standing in line at a store, he heard the squeal of vehicle tires and smelled burning rubber. "I began to shake. My heart was racing, and my palms were sweating. I started hyperventilating," David recalled. He left the line, grabbed a bottle of Jack Daniels whiskey, opened it, and took a long swig.

"I thought, 'Okay, well that takes care of that.' So every time that feeling would creep up, I'd go drink."

David was honorably discharged from the Army in 2005. He described his life after the war as an escape from reality. His nervous system couldn't handle noise. A car backfiring brought on the jitters and sweats. His language at home was coarse and unwelcome. His behavior was so erratic that his parents literally felt that their son might harm them.

His life began to change when he heard a radio advertisement. A study was being conducted on the benefits of Transcendental Meditation for veterans suffering from combat stress and post-traumatic stress disorder. The advertisement offered to teach TM to those who qualified and enrolled in the study. David applied and was accepted.

As David describes it, he finally found something that gave him relief. "The first time I meditated, I experienced this relief from the constant anxiety attack my life had become. I didn't even realize I was that stressed out until after my first 20-minute meditation. I was like, 'That was a break.' I realized that this is what my life could become—life that wasn't constantly being tormented by this horrible uncontrollable feeling, this constant anxiety attack that my life was then. When I meditated, it stopped. I just felt completely relaxed for the first time in five years. I didn't even realize how wound up I'd become."

Like David, Dan Burks was an Army

Infantryman. His service was during the Vietnam War—a different war but a similar story.

"My dad was in World War II, Normandy, the Battle of the Bulge," Dan explained. "I had a scholarship to go to college. I went for one year. Everybody was there to avoid the draft. At the end of the year I thought, 'No, this is wrong. I'm gonna go to war. That's what my family does.'"

Dan volunteered for the Infantry. He wanted to be part of the Airborne, but he wore glasses. So he memorized the eye chart. At his vision test he screened as 20/40 vision. From then on he always made sure he had three pairs of glasses with him at all times.

Once in Vietnam, Dan ended up as a machine gunner. One night in Bu Dop, his unit was attacked. He recalled the experience: "That fight went on for two weeks. The first night I killed fourteen people. There were 2,500 of them, and 250 of us. And we kicked their butt. Then, the next morning, in front of my fighting position on the airstrip, 18 of our men lay dead. *(Long pause)* This was very, very, very distressing. It creates huge amounts of distress in your system. There's no way to relieve the stress.

"So everybody's smoking pot to cope," Dan explained.

"And then you go home.

"All these people don't understand you. They have no idea. They don't realize that you're always, always still in the rubber plantation, in the jungle. You're always on an adrenaline high. You're looking to do things: looking to protect your buddies, looking to protect yourself, looking to kill the enemy. You've got to do your job.

"I couldn't get along with other people, and pretty soon I stopped talking to my parents. Things were going to shit. I was not the same person."

Dan returned to school, trying to return to the life he had before Vietnam. But he couldn't concentrate. He would sit in class, but he just couldn't focus. He couldn't walk in the woods, which he used to love doing, because he was always looking for an ambush. "There was no way to stop," he says. "It's an internal thing. It's a mind-body-spirit-nervous system— everything.

"I had no feelings. I did not feel happiness. I did not feel sorrow. I did not feel surprise. My feelings were gone."

One day Dan's wife saw a poster for Transcendental Meditation. (Thank heaven for those who love and support us.) Being a good Infantryman, Dan sent in a scout—his wife Cindy. She learned first. Dan remembers it well: "I could not believe it. I could not believe what she looked like. She was glowing, just glowing. So I said, okay, I'll go do this.

"When I learned, I could not believe what happened. It was the difference between heaven and hell. It was absolutely transformational. All that feeling of stress, and all that feeling of heaviness, I could feel it melt it away, from my head to my feet.

"And from that moment on, things changed. Things changed big time. No more drugs, no more alcohol. Life changed. My emotions came back. My life came back. As time went on, I stopped looking for ambushes. I was able to go back out in the woods, which I really enjoy. My wife and I got along better. All of a sudden my parents were back. I started making friends again. My grades went back up to A's. Sex was better. Everything was just better."

Chapter 6:
Connections

When I talk with these veterans, I am struck with how similar all of our experiences were after we returned home. There is a powerful feeling of being an outsider, of not fitting in, a feeling that no one understands you or knows what you went through. It's hard to talk to civilians. In the military culture, with your buddies, every paragraph is punctuated with the F-word. It's a verb, it's a noun, and it's a strong affirmative when expressed with emphasis as "F—in' A." Out of the military, your language seems inappropriate and harsh.

Ron Khare, a Vietnam veteran, describes it this way, "I was hard, solid. I had nothing. I was dead. I was walking dead. The only thing that kept me going was respect for those who didn't make it. It was not acceptable for me to disappear when those guys would have liked to have been there."

Ron joined the Marines right out of high school. After boot camp he was sent to Vietnam. He was not on the front line — as he puts it, "just a guy in the rear with the gear." But he saw the tragedies of war. His friends were maimed and killed. And then he was discharged, and returned home to civilian life.

His friends from home tried to help. Their advice: "You've got a problem? Have a shot. Get drunk like everybody else. Drink yourself blind every night. That's what real men do. Don't go bellyaching, 'Oh, you have flashbacks and bad dreams' — everyone has them.'"

Or when he'd tell people about his experiences, they would say "Oh, that was a long time ago. Forget it. Get over it."

You don't get over it. You can't get over it. Today they call it post-traumatic stress disorder, but when Ron came back from Vietnam it didn't have a name. The military members who suffer from these hidden wounds of war do not get Purple Hearts. And so you look for an escape—alcohol, marijuana, prescription drugs—anything to dull the pain, the memories that we veterans do not speak about.

Chapter 7:
Healing

What is this thing that has changed the lives of those of us who tell our stories in this book? The Transcendental Meditation technique is a simple, natural, mental procedure. It's easy to learn, and easy to do. You do it twice a day for 15 to 20 minutes each time, sitting comfortably with the eyes closed. The technique turns the attention inward to experience deeper levels of thought, until you go beyond active thought, and the mind comes to a state of complete inner rest. But the mind is alert; it's not like being asleep. There is an inner wakefulness, and a feeling of calm and peace.

It's a unique experience.

It makes sense that a meditation technique can help with recovery from combat stress or post-traumatic stress disorder (PTSD). After all, it is called post-traumatic *stress*.

But PTSD isn't garden-variety stress. It's not like the stress of having a project report due or sitting in rush hour traffic. The trauma of battle, seeing friends wounded and killed, creates intense stress.

David George, the Iraq veteran I spoke of earlier in the book, describes driving up to a stop sign at night near his home. "It was dark. I was stopped; in my mind I was a sitting target."

Brenda Marlin, also an Iraq veteran and on active duty now at the Pentagon, says, "You can't explain the reaction every time you see a box or trashcan on the street. Automatically you start thinking, 'Is this an IED? Is it going to explode?'"

PTSD is different from a normal stress response because the symptoms continue long after the cause of the stress or fear is gone. This type of stressful event creates such a strong impression in the mind that it takes very little to activate the memory to such a high degree that the experience seems real again.   A reflexive reaction takes over, bypassing the intellect and logic that might tell you it's not real, you're somewhere else, and there is no threat.

In the normal stress response, the brain floods with adrenaline.   The lungs pump faster, and the heart starts to race.   Blood pressure rises, stimulating the muscles and sharpening the mind on a single reference point—the stressor.   The stomach gets "jumpy," and the release of endorphins numbs the body.   Appetite, libido, and the immune system shut down.   All the energy normally directed to these functions is redirected to the muscles.   This is the "fight-or-flight" response. It's this response that gives you the strength to do the heroic job you have to do, or run for help as fast as you can.   Once stress is removed, life returns to normal.

The ability to achieve stability through change is critical to survival.   But the price of this constant response to stress can be overload, causing wear and tear to the nervous system. Over time, stress and the continuing physiological response to it can become debilitating. The system breaks down.

This kind of stress causes changes in the mind and body that easily trigger the fight-or-flight response, even when it's not needed. The brain chemistry is actually altered. Disruption in these systems can cause hypervigilence, like that described by David and Brenda. This helps explain the startle reflex, such as jumping to reach for a weapon when you hear a loud noise. It's the source of "re-experiencing," reliving the event in your mind, triggered by similar images, sounds, or smells. It becomes hard to control an anger response. Something is way out of whack in the system.

What happens is that chronic stress, constantly being in the fight-or-flight response mode, being ready to "do your job" 24 hours a day, recalibrates your body, and you can't get back to your baseline. You can't bounce back to normal. The resilience is gone.

But Transcendental Meditation can help

restore the resilience. TM creates a response that is the opposite of the stress response. During TM the mind settles down to a state of restful alertness. As the mind settles down, the body becomes deeply relaxed. As the thinking process continues to refine through the technique, the mind transcends, or goes beyond mental activity, and you experience deep silence. This produces a unique fourth state of consciousness—"Transcendental Consciousness"—described by researchers as a state of "restful alertness." In this state, the mind is alert, while the body is deeply relaxed.

The heart rate slows down, breathing slows and becomes shallower, blood pressure lowers, and the flow of blood to the arms and legs is reduced—similar to how the body is during sleep. But you're not asleep. Both the mind and body are relaxed. That feeling begins to stay with you after meditation. And it lasts longer and longer until finally it replaces the debilitating feelings of anxiety and stress for good.

Chapter 8:
Women in Service

The role of women in the military has expanded considerably in recent years and now includes combat-related roles. Like their male peers, women are dedicated and courageous in their service. But women in the military face greater challenges, both in service and when they return home. There is constant pressure to prove to themselves, and to others, that they can survive and excel in this "man's world." They have to overcome the biases that can still persist in the military: the notion that women are weaker, more fearful, and less competent than men.

When they return home from service, the challenges for women continue to be greater than for their male counterparts. Being away for months at a time, often with multiple deployments, puts a strain on the families of both men and women. And all too often the return home adds even greater strain as the serviceman or woman tries to reintegrate into the family, while also trying to adjust to life outside a war zone. As a result, the divorce rate among the military has steadily increased over the last three years. But it is the military women who have been most affected. The divorce rate among military women is a staggering three times higher than that of men.

Brenda Marlinbanks is an Army Reserve Lieutenant Colonel with twenty-seven years of commissioned service and eight years of enlisted service. She was attending the Joint Air Commanders Course at Hurlbert Field in Florida when America was attacked on 9/11. After the invasion of Iraq her reserve unit was mobilized and sent to Qatar to support OIF/OEF (Operation Iraqi Freedom and Operation Enduring Freedom in Afghanistan).

She was the only female to deploy with thirty-eight men from her unit. Fortunately she was accustomed by then to being the only female, and likewise the guys were comfortable with her, too. She had proven herself.

"My lodging at the female officers' quarters was a large, unoccupied, general purpose tent. Another female lieutenant colonel and I were the sole occupants. We brought our own gear: foldout sleeping cots, rolled mats and sleeping bags, and duffle bags full of other gear and personal items, including makeup," Brenda recalled.

During her deployment she spent ten months in Qatar in unimaginable temperatures and sandstorms, doing duty shifts of twelve hours or more daily. She was responsible for coordinating battlefield activities and air strike support. This included constant vigilance for suspicious activities, events, and people; keeping track of all IED attacks; and documenting friendly and enemy/insurgent killed or wounded in action.

She was vigilantly alert—constantly aware that an IED could be anything, anybody, and anywhere.   In addition to pedestrians and motor vehicles carrying IEDs, explosives were planted on bicycles, wheelchairs, goat carts, market venders, animal carcasses, roadside signs, live donkeys, just about anything.

"Returning home was a welcome relief, but it brought new unanticipated stress," Brenda remembers. "First of all, I had not done any cooking, household chores, gone anywhere without my gear, or worn civilian clothes (except on rare occasions) for almost a year. I was uncomfortable in open places, didn't like being in traffic, and was suspicious of delivery trucks and crews. The war theater had become my comfort zone, and I missed it. I missed the routine, and I missed my crew. My civilian life seemed frivolous and meaningless."

Thirteen months after her return, Brenda was mobilized for OIF/OEF support at the Pentagon, serving three years on the Joint Staff and two years on the Army Staff, becoming team chief at the National Military Command Center.

"We were all stressed over casualty counts and the many variables in the war. At some point my mind became really cluttered, and I realized I was having difficulty concentrating. I became a marathon runner. It really helped me relax, but didn't do anything to improve my focus. I talked to several coworkers who were basically going through the same thing. So I concluded that this was my new normal, and I'd just have to deal with it."

Brenda pushed on, completing the Air Force War College and the National Defense University's Advance Joint Professional Military Education II (AJPME), while working fulltime at the Pentagon. About midway through AJPME, she suffered a ruptured aneurysm, underwent two brain surgeries, and still managed to finish AJPME on time with her class.

During all this, her marriage began to fall apart. And then she found out she had breast cancer. Under the stress of her military duties, her illness, and a marriage that was falling apart, she couldn't sleep and couldn't focus. She started to think she was having a nervous breakdown.

"I spoke with a psychiatrist who told me my mental and emotional states were excellent, but suggested relaxation techniques. I discussed this with a friend (an Air Force officer), and she described how Transcendental Meditation had helped her. Of course, I was skeptical. It just seemed too wimpy for an Army person. But I trusted her advice. I knew she had gone through some personal difficulties and was coping very well. So I decided to try it, and I'm grateful that I did.

"Just a few days after I began TM, I was able to sort through all the loose thoughts and tasks that were fogging up my mind. TM gave me clarity to prioritize the important things and discard the junk that was eating up a lot of precious time. Now I have more time, and feel less anxious and stressed.

"The calm I get from meditation has improved my memory and my ability to concentrate.   I am more focused and settled. I'm sleeping better and longer, and feel less anxious throughout the day.   It's hard to believe that something so simple could be so effective, and so fast."

Chapter 9:
Soldier's Reflections

Lieutenant Colonel Allan Long[1] served in Afghanistan as part of the 82nd Airborne. He was a strong leader who represented all that the 82nd stands for. "I never took a sick day. I wanted to be a role model for my troops," he told me. Two years after retiring from the Army, Allan was diagnosed with PTSD. "Now I realize I should have set the example that you need to take care of yourself—get help when you need it."

The mentality of "Army Strong," and the equivalent in the other services, has made it difficult for any warrior to acknowledge that he or she needs help—much less to seek that help. Despite legislation passed by the U.S. Congress to de-stigmatize combat stress, presentations made to troops when they return

---

[1] Name has been changed to protect privacy.

home, and speaking tours given by high-level military leaders, it is still very difficult to overcome a culture that has been ingrained in the fabric of the military for generations. This is a culture that views a problem, especially problems of the mind, as weakness.

For many the fear of being perceived weak is so strong that some choose to take their own life rather than let others know they are suffering. The consequences are devastating to their families, their buddies, and to the military, which is struggling to figure out how to identify and help those who are quietly fighting their own inner war.

Ft. Hood, which has struggled with a dramatic number of suicides, recently conducted a confidential survey to discover the soldiers' views about seeking help. Twenty-five percent of the respondents said they would be viewed as weak, treated differently, or would damage their careers if they admitted suffering with emotional issues and/or problems. That attitude was particularly strong among majors, lieutenant colonels, and full colonels. It is evident that, aside from the leaders in the Pentagon who seek solutions, this is a view that pervades the military from the top down.

Even those who are no longer in the service feel the burden of this stigma. Aaron Green[2] retired from the Army as a 1st Sergeant after twenty-two years, serving combat tours in Bosnia, Iraq, and two tours in Afghanistan. He described his experience this way: "It's not been easy for me acknowledging that I have symptoms of post-traumatic stress disorder. I realize now that these symptoms were causing me to be a liability in day-to-day activities at home and work. I believe I clearly have PTSD, but will never mention it to the VA. If I do let others know, I believe there will be discrimination.

"Some things that were always racing in my mind were emotions, anxiety, depression,

---

[2] Name has been changed to protect privacy.

insomnia at times, problems communicating with others, and anger. These bad traits were causing family problems and were very uncomfortable, to say the least. It's a scary feeling to possibly have these things throwing my quality of life out of balance.

"My biggest fear with these problems was becoming unemployed and unmarketable in the workforce. I believe if you were to whisper any of these symptoms—being a retired soldier—it would mean certain unemployment and loss of security clearance immediately."

Aaron found a confidential and private resource for overcoming these problems. "This will be my third month practicing Transcendental Meditation, and I can say for me it has been vastly effective.

"Transcendental Meditation has given me the needed assistance to take back control of my emotions and thoughts that were starting to make me dysfunctional as a family member and a part of society. I wasn't functioning to my full potential prior to TM, and now I am back to a normal way of life.

"Since I have been practicing TM daily, I now feel relaxed at the beginning of the day, orderly and ready for the day, and project a positive vibe to others at work. I'm more cognitive, and think clearly before acting on certain things.

"I can completely unwind at the end of the day. Thoughts of previous events that were disturbing and causing problems are less detailed. I'm thankful for what I have and where I am at in my life.

"Bottom line: TM has given me the opportunity to regain and start rebuilding my physical health and mental well- being. It is a new way for me to treat problems myself mentally, instead of using the conventional method of medication or acting out."

Chapter 10:
TM for Healing

Family and friends are often among those who suffer most from the collateral damage when a service person, scarred from his or her experiences, returns home. "My wife left and took the kids," said Ted Swanson,[3] a Marine veteran from the Iraq War. "Within the first few days after learning TM, I felt like a lot of weight was taken off my shoulders." Today Ted is back with his wife and children. TM helped him control his anger, reduce his hypervigilence, feel emotion again, and allow his happiness to extend to his family.

"When I got back, I didn't feel a part of society. I just self-medicated with alcohol and went into isolation, stopped seeing friends," says Jeff Larson,[4] a Gulf War veteran and

---

[3] Name has been changed to protect privacy.

[4] Name has been changed to protect privacy.

contractor in Iraq. "TM allowed me to find that peace and release the stress."

But what about those memories that show up unexpectedly like a freight train barreling through your thoughts when some sound or smell takes you back to its source? Every experience changes the brain. When an experience is repeated the neural pathways of the brain get strengthened. For example, when a star quarterback like Payton Manning first started throwing a football, his brain connections were there. But through practice of throwing a football over and over again, his speed of mental processing, hand-eye coordination, and agility got better and better. That happens because the circuits in the brain, the thought processes that orchestrate the action and send the signals about throwing, got thicker and faster.

Soldiers in combat re-experience stressful events over and over again. This has the potential to imbed the stressful memories in the same way an athlete's activity is imbedded in his brain. Conventional wisdom says that you eventually get used to the memories and they stop affecting you in the same way. Eventually you stop breaking out in a sweat, your heart stops pounding, and your blood pressure doesn't go up every time you're in a crowd or you come to a stop sign on a deserted corner at night.

Maybe that works. But maybe it doesn't. It would be better to override those stressful memories with something more pleasant, to strengthen the brain connections associated with feeling good. Then that experience will dominate. With Transcendental Meditation twice a day, the brain experiences inner silence: Your thinking mind goes beyond the boundaries of a thought to experience unbounded awareness, your own inner self. This experience strengthens the brain circuitry associated with happiness. With the regular practice of TM, that circuitry becomes stronger and stronger. It's much like working out. You go to the gym to develop strength and endurance. When you work out regularly, that strength and endurance stays with you all the time. TM is like exercise for the brain. The great thing is, it's effortless—you do it with your eyes closed!

You know the expression "use it or lose it." When you regularly activate the brain circuitry that creates feelings of happiness, stability, and freedom, those experiences predominate, and the unpleasant memories start to weaken. They never go away, but they fade far into the background. And this happens naturally and spontaneously, not by dulling the mind with drugs or alcohol.

Some of the stories presented in this chapter come from participants in a recent research study. This study measured the presence and degree of war trauma–related symptoms in Iraq and Afghanistan veterans before learning TM and after practicing the technique for some time. The majority of the participants experienced 50 percent less PTSD symptoms by the fourth week of meditating, and even greater improvements after two months and three months. These included reduced symptoms of re-experiencing, hyper-vigilance, avoidance, memory problems, and emotional numbness. Depression was reduced, and quality of life increased, based on the objective assessments. In a short time, the participants saw very big changes. As one subject described it, "If you want to be who you really are, do TM, and go ahead and live again."

That research was a pilot study, the first study of TM with veterans from the Iraq/Afghanistan wars. Though it did not have a large number of subjects, and there was no comparison group (more complete studies are now in the works), the results are corroborated by a control-group study with Vietnam veterans, conducted in the mid-1980s. In that study, participating veterans at a Colorado Vet Center were randomly assigned to either a group that would learn TM or a group that would receive standard psychotherapy. After three months, the group practicing the TM technique had statistically significant reductions in PTSD symptoms of emotional numbness, anxiety, startle response, depression, alcohol consumption, and family problems. The psychotherapy group had little, if any, improvement. It was also reported that the TM group had significant improvements in sleep, and in obtaining/keeping employment. Seventy percent of the TM group reported that they no longer needed the services of the Vet Center.

Almost all of the veterans I've talked with say that at some point they self-medicated with alcohol or drugs, looking for some way to stop their anxiety, stress, or pain. During the course of learning TM, there is no instruction or admonition about cigarette smoking or drinking. Everyone has his or her own lifestyle, and TM doesn't require any change in that.

Yet studies show decreases in alcohol and drug use after learning TM. Studies also show that 50 percent of cigarette smokers who learned TM stopped smoking, and were still not smoking nineteen months later. A typical success rate for smoking cessation programs specifically designed to help someone quit smoking is about 15 percent. An analysis of the effectiveness of various smoking cessation techniques found that TM is twice as effective as any other approach. But the interesting thing is that it happens naturally as a side benefit of TM practice.

Chapter 11:
Affect of TM on PTSD

PTSD doesn't just affect the mind. People who suffer the symptoms of PTSD also have a higher risk of heart disease and autoimmune diseases such as arthritis, diabetes, psoriasis, and thyroid disease. So it's logical that reducing or eliminating the symptoms of PTSD will improve your health over time. Transcendental Meditation not only improves mental and physical health by reducing the symptoms of PTSD; it improves overall health, boosts the immune system, and improves psychological wellbeing.

Many published studies, most funded by the National Institutes of Health (NIH), have shown the effectiveness of TM for reducing high blood pressure, reducing the risk of heart attack and stroke, and even reversing the progression of heart disease. (Instead of blood vessels continuing to get thicker and thicker with blockage over time, TM resulted in reduction of blockage.)

Since stress complicates or is an associated cause of up to 90 percent of all illness, it is clear how TM can improve overall health. A number of studies have been done using data from national insurance companies that compare health care use and costs between TM meditators and non-meditators. The data show that, on average, TM meditators have 50 percent fewer visits to the doctor, 50 percent less hospital visits and shorter hospital stays, and a 50 percent reduction in health care costs. Those are average reductions for all medical reasons. For heart disease, the reductions are an astounding 87 percent.

Just in case you're thinking that people who meditate are "alternative types," and probably don't like doctors and don't see them when they are sick, the research shows no statistical difference between meditator and non-meditator use of obstetric services and hospital admissions for childbirth. That means meditators use health care services, when needed, as much as the next person. They are just generally healthier and therefore have a dramatically lower need for health care.

There are several studies showing that TM meditators live longer than non-meditators.

One I find especially interesting is a recent study that followed a group with existing heart disease over a nine-year period. There were, of course, significant reductions in psychological stress among the meditators. But this also translated into a 47 percent reduction in the combination of death, heart attacks, and strokes in the TM group. This study shows the value of the long-term practice of TM in reducing your risk of dying from a heart attack or stroke.

Though the data did not reach statistical significance, TM has also been shown to lower the risk of dying of cancer by 49 percent. So just sitting, closing the eyes for 20 minutes and doing TM can dramatically increase your longevity!

Chapter 12:
Peak Performing Warriors

You may be asking yourself how meditation might fit into the military culture. But the question we should be asking is how meditation got separated from the military culture. If we think back through history to the greatest example of a finely tuned warrior, it would have to be the Japanese samurai. The training of a samurai warrior was centered on "union." An expert samurai represented the total integration, the total union, of mind and body—quick, clear thinking, combined with precision and strength of the body, working as one.

The intimate connection between mind and body is lost in military training today. Today, we train the warrior's mind by filling it with information about how to respond to every imaginable situation, and we train the body in strength and endurance. But we train them separately. Then we provide strong protective armor for the body, but nothing for the mind.

To add to the problem, at a time of extreme stress or crisis (which is essentially every minute of the day in a combat environment), the connection between the mind and the body sometimes breaks down totally.

Under stress, the fight-or-flight response takes over. There is a rush of adrenaline, and all the energy goes to the muscles. The part of the brain that is responsible for clear thinking—analysis, logic, planning, and organization—just switches off. What takes over is the emotional or reactive part of the brain. So the body performs almost by reflex, disconnected from thinking.

In this situation all the information, intellectual training, and role-playing practice goes out the window. The mind and body are no longer synchronized. The body is acting, and the mind is in panic. Nature has given us this mechanism to survive. The body gives its all, sometimes miraculously, to create safety any way it can. But when the body reacts without the guidance of the brain, mistakes are made, opportunities are lost, and the outcome can be worse than it should have been.

The Transcendental Meditation technique is thousands of years old, highly prized by the military throughout time. TM creates the union between mind and body. TM provides a means of connecting with the solid foundation that is our own inner core of strength, establishing us in the unbounded field that is the source of everything, where everything is unified.

When we access this source, it actually affects brain functioning. The brain becomes highly coherent. This means that all the different parts of the brain—right and left hemisphere, front of the brain and rear of the brain—are functioning together, unified in processing the data necessary for action. Usually when we engage in a particular task, for example finding a location on a map, very specific parts of the brain are called into action. When we do other types of activities, such as driving an armored vehicle, other parts of the brain are performing.

During TM, the entire brain works together as one.   This whole-brain functioning then continues after meditation, during daily activity. The result is the ability to draw on the full potential of brain power: analysis, visual-motor coordination, planning, action, big picture, fine details, and emotion, all together, such that maximum brain power is brought to the task.

This is peak performance.   In fact, a research study compared brain functioning of elite, medal-winning Olympic athletes to that of non-athletes who were TM meditators. The medal winners talked about being "in the zone" during peak performance. This union of mind and body has a unique pattern of measurable brain waves. What is remarkable is that the coherent brain functioning of the meditators was the same as that of the elite athletes when they were in the zone. The athletes had to train rigorously, long and hard; while the pattern of whole-brain functioning developed spontaneously for the meditators just from their TM practice.

If the body is trained for peak performance, and the mind is drawn back to its source of inner strength through meditation, the connection of mind and body results in a finely tuned warrior who is resilient and clear thinking under stress. He or she becomes an optimum leader who exemplifies peak performance. That is the model warrior.

Recently I met a retired Army officer. He confided to me that when he returned from Vietnam in 1972 he felt lost. He entered the Army language school but couldn't concentrate, felt he was in over his head, and quickly fell behind. He was struggling, adrift, and even contemplated suicide.

He saw an advertisement for Transcendental Meditation and decided to learn. Very quickly he regained his footing.

He felt better, happier, able to concentrate, and he rapidly caught up with his classmates. He went on to have a long and productive career in the Army, eventually serving a critical role in overseeing the military communication structure for the Iraq war until he retired as a Lieutenant Colonel three years ago. He practiced TM throughout his military career.

This man's service career could have been tragically cut short. But by discovering and learning TM he became a critical asset to the military, retiring proudly after a fulfilling service to his country. Today he serves on the board of a prestigious veteran's organization, continues to contribute to the service of his country, and still does TM every day.

Richard Sullivan[5] was a Marine who served in Vietnam. on several tours of duty. When he came home on permanent assignment he became a division leader, a commander.

Richard was experiencing more stress than

---

[5] Name has been changed to protect privacy.

he had ever known, and more than he wanted to acknowledge. He was athletic, so he turned to strenuous workouts as a means of relieving the stress. It helped, but the stress still continued to build up.

Richard had also been fascinated by the idea of strengthening not only his body but also his mind and spirit. Then in 1977 he read about Transcendental Meditation and decided to learn to meditate. Within three weeks he saw a noticeable change. He felt a psychological and emotional calmness that he hadn't experienced before. "When I worked out before I learned to meditate, I felt good, in shape and alert. But after I learned TM it was different. My mind was sharper; I was more open, my thoughts were clearer, more composed," Richard told me. "When I ran or worked out, it could clear out some of the cobwebs, but TM does more than that. It gives me a real sense of comfort."

Richard retired from the Marines in 1997 as a Lieutenant Colonel.

Peak performance and strong leadership are the qualities of excellence in a military professional. This takes a settled mind, quick thinking, broad vision, confidence in your decisions, and resilience. The most damaging influence on these qualities is stress.

The greatest weapon in a military professional's arsenal is the mind. The most efficient and effective technique for developing a sharp mind is the Transcendental Meditation technique.

Dan Burks, whose story I recounted in Chapter 5, expresses what so many warriors feel—that the desire to serve never goes away. But there is more to Dan's story. In 1978, several years after he learned TM and, as he said, "my life came back," Dan was in graduate school. The chairman of his academic department was a Colonel in military intelligence in the reserves. One day he said to Dan, "Why don't you join the reserves?"

Dan's reaction: "You've got to be kidding me. There's no way."

"Come on," encouraged the chairman, "You can do it. Come on. Be in my unit. It's fun. You like to read books."

So Dan signed up for ROTC. And a year later he was in the Infantry again, this time as an officer.

"But what had gone away," Dan tells me, "was the stress." Dan ended up serving twenty years. But now he was also a TM meditator. He remembers the difference: "My reaction time was better. I was more adaptable. I was more creative. I was better with my men, way better. And they respected me more."

Chapter 13:
Comparison of Meditation Techniques

By now you may be feeling that meditation could be the missing piece to creating a whole warrior. But you also might be asking yourself, "Does it really matter what type of meditation I do?" Since TM was introduced in the U.S. by Maharishi Mahesh Yogi over fifty years ago, dozens of meditation and self-help techniques have sprouted up. Is TM any different or any better than the others?

Once again, we can turn to science. When the first research was conducted on the Transcendental Meditation technique in the early 1970s, there was a common hypothesis that all techniques of meditation and relaxation would reduce stress and produce similar changes in the nervous system—and therefore all techniques should be equally effective. For many researchers and doctors, this proposal soon became accepted as fact. But this hypothesis has not withstood the test of scientific scrutiny. In fact, it has been shown that some meditation techniques actually increase stress.

Different types of meditation, relaxation, and mental techniques involve different mechanics, different types of mental activity. Therefore it can be expected that different techniques will affect the mind and body in uniquely different ways.

A meta-analysis is a study that combines the results of several studies to determine the effectiveness of approaches. A meta-analysis was used to compare the effectiveness of various relaxation techniques for reducing anxiety. One hundred and forty-six studies were analyzed—virtually all of the published research that met basic design criteria at the time. The studies were grouped according to the type of relaxation technique used and the number of studies in each category.

All techniques were found to be equal to or *less* effective than placebo (that is, they were no better than doing nothing), with the exception of Transcendental Meditation. TM was shown to be almost two and half times more effective than any other technique. The study also showed that meditations involving concentration led to an *increase* in anxiety, further emphasizing that not all meditation techniques yield the same results.

A recently published study compared the brain patterns during different meditation techniques. The study showed that TM produces a distinctively different brain pattern from that of the other techniques. The study quantified the experience of transcending the active, noisy level of thinking, to experience the infinite silence of your own conscious awareness. And it happens without effort. This is referred to as "automatic self-transcending."

The combination of the uniqueness of brain functioning during TM practice and the substantial research showing its greater effectiveness compared to other techniques puts Transcendental Meditation in a category of its own.

Chapter 14:
The Resilient Warrior

What makes the current wars in Iraq and Afghanistan so difficult for our troops? War is always difficult for those on the front lines, but these two wars are being fought in the countries of our enemies, on their territory, in their homeland, their cities. And there are no established front lines or objectives to capture. Every citizen can be looked at as "the enemy," every road as a dangerous road to travel, every pile of garbage as a possible IED ready to explode.

In the book The Three Trillion Dollar War, written by Joseph E. Stiglitz, Nobel Laureate, and Linda L. Bilmes, a Harvard professor, we get a glimpse of the different realities between World War II and the wars in Iraq and Afghanistan.

There were 16 million service people in World War II and 385,000 were killed. The ratio of wounded to killed was 1:6—one wounded for every six killed.

According to the statistics compiled by the Department of Veterans Affairs in 2006, the ratio of 7 wounded to each death in Iraq and Afghanistan is startling, 7:1. Then if you added to these numbers those who became ill while in a combat zone, the staggering number of casualties to deaths reaches 15:1.

As I write this, 5,745 of our servicemen and women have been killed, and 86,175 have been evacuated for wounds or illness: 21.7% of the approximately 2 million who have seen active duty.

It has been estimated that 35 to 40% of those who have served since 2003 suffer from post-traumatic stress disorder. Since the average age of the current military is 21, these veterans could require care for 50 or 60 years or more. The cost to care for our veterans, as estimated by Stiglitz and Bilmes, is $5,765 per veteran per year—or a total that could reach $717 billion just to service the estimated 2.1 million veterans of Iraq and Afghanistan. This estimate does not take into account additional costs to the government for benefits to the families of wounded and mentally ill veterans. Every veteran who is wounded or mentally ill adversely affects everyone in his or her household. The entire family suffers and has needs.

If my story and the stories of others told in this book can serve as examples of recovery from PTSD, it is self-evident that Transcendental Meditation should be offered as an option to all veterans. The cost per veteran to learn TM—for a lifetime of health—is just one quarter of the projected cost to the Veterans Administration for treatment for one year.

Even better would be to offer Transcendental Meditation to every individual who enters the military, to create a well-rounded warrior with a clear and settled mind, one who is quick thinking, has broad vision, confidence, and can perform at the highest level as a Resilient Warrior.

Chapter 15:
The Transcendental Meditation Technique

Questions and Answers

What is Transcendental Meditation?

The Transcendental Meditation technique is simple, natural, effortless, and easily learned. It is practiced for 20 minutes twice a day while sitting comfortably with the eyes closed. The TM technique is not a religion or philosophy, nor does it require any change of lifestyle. It is taught by a certified TM teacher through a seven-step course of instruction.

The TM course is followed by weekly, and then monthly, checking sessions (averaging 20–30 minutes) to ensure correct practice of the technique. The course also includes an optional, lifetime follow-up of checking and knowledge to ensure maximum benefit. Anyone 10 years of age or older can learn the practice. (There's a special technique for children under 10.)

Can I learn the TM technique from a book?

The TM technique is unique among forms of meditation. It's natural and effortless, but requires personal instruction to learn. Imagine trying to learn a natural golf stroke from a book. Or if you have ever learned to play a musical instrument, you know how helpful it is to have a good teacher. The teacher is needed to show you proper technique so that you can grow in confidence that you're proceeding along correctly. Learning the TM technique is a lot easier than mastering the piano or getting a good, natural golf swing, but involves the same kind of personalized guidance.

How does the TM technique work?

Deep within the mind of every human being is a field of pure wakefulness, a field of lively silence. This is the quiet, inner source of energy, creativity, and intelligence within everyone. But most of us don't notice it because we are constantly wrapped up in the noisy activity of our world.

The TM technique allows anyone to effortlessly access this inner field of restful alertness. This is a soothing and healing experience; more than 600 scientific studies, published in top medical journals, have documented improvement in almost every area of life through practicing the Transcendental Meditation technique.

What if I can't sit still to meditate?

The experience of restful alertness is pleasant and comfortable, and this allows you to continue to sit quietly for twenty minutes twice a day. When practiced regularly, this program dissolves stress cumulatively, and with time, you experience less and less stress and nervousness. As a natural result of this lessening of stress, the mind settles down when you're meditating and you don't feel the need to get up and move around. The direct experience of stillness and peace takes care of those feelings of restlessness.

With continued practice, anxiety plays less and less a role in a person's life; the individual starts making better decisions about daily activities because he or she is better able to cope with stress. So, with time, one gains the possibility of becoming stress free. This means being motivated by the needs of the situation rather than one's own stressful response to the situation. Instead of reacting to challenges as a threat, one sees challenges as an opportunity for personal and professional growth.

Is TM the same as relaxing?

Not according to the science. A wide range of beneficial physiological changes commonly occur during Transcendental Meditation practice, changes that distinguish the technique from mere relaxation and other forms of meditation. Studies indicate that TM practice produces a state of rest much deeper than sitting with eyes closed, and also much deeper than other meditation practices. Research consistently shows a natural decrease in breath rate during the TM technique, 25 percent greater than non-meditating control groups, and an increase in basal skin resistance (a standard measure of relaxation) up to 70 percent higher.

Physiological indicators of deep rest also include marked changes in respiratory volume, minute ventilation, tidal volume, blood lactate, and heart rate. Studies suggest that this unique state of physiological functioning helps regulate cortisol and other hormones associated with chronic stress—and also promotes healthier regulation of serotonin, a neurotransmitter associated with mood.

Even more significant, measurement of brain waves shows increased integration and orderliness of brain functioning—further differentiating the Transcendental Meditation technique from ordinary relaxation and other meditation practices.

Is TM a religion—or does it require any specific belief or lifestyle?

TM is not a religion or philosophy, and involves no change in lifestyle. You can even be skeptical that it will work, and it will still work.

So how do you learn TM?

TM is taught by certified teachers. The initial phase of TM instruction can be mastered in seven simple steps during which the technique is learned very systematically through the alternation of direct experience and additional personal instruction. The course takes a total of about ten hours over 4–5 days (about 1.5 hours per day). After these seven steps have been completed, new meditators may take advantage of further opportunities to ensure correct practice of the technique and also to gain more understanding of the practice through highly engaging follow-up seminars.

The Transcendental Meditation Technique

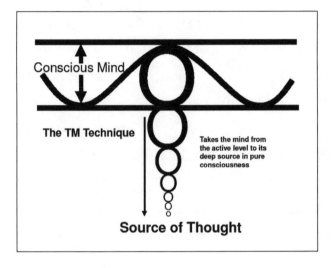

Conscious Mind

The TM Technique

Takes the mind from the active level to its deep source in pure consciousness

Source of Thought

The Transcendental Meditation technique turns the attention inward to experience deeper levels of thought, until you go beyond active thought and the mind comes to a state of complete inner rest.   But the mind is alert. There is an inner wakefulness, and a feeling of calm and peace.   This is a state of *restful alertness*. The brain functions with significantly greater coherence and your body gains deep rest.

Physiological Indicators of Deep Rest During the Transcendental Meditation Technique

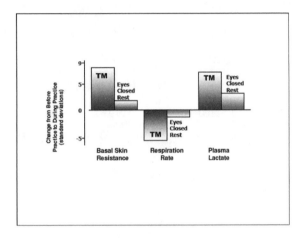

During the practice of the Transcendental Meditation technique the body settles into deep rest. The heart rate slows down, breathing slows and becomes shallower, blood pressure lowers, and the flow of blood to the arms and legs is reduced – similar to how the body is during sleep. Both the mind and body are relaxed, but the mind is alert. This is a state of restful alertness.

Dillbeck MC, Orme-Johnson DW. Physiological differences between Transcendental Meditation and rest. *American Psychologist* 1987 42(9):879–881

Effects of Transcendental Meditation on Iraq and Afghanistan War Veterans with Post-Traumatic Stress

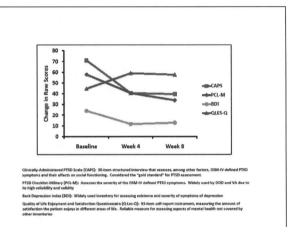

Clinically-Administered PTSD Scale (CAPS): 30-item structured interview that assesses, among other factors, DSM-IV defined PTSD symptoms and their effects on social functioning. Considered the "gold standard" for PTSD assessment.

PTSD Checklist-Military (PCL-M): Assesses the severity of the DSM-IV defined PTSD symptoms. Widely used by DOD and VA due to its high reliability and validity

Beck Depression Index (BDI): Widely used inventory for assessing existence and severity of symptoms of depression

Quality of Life Enjoyment and Satisfaction Questionnaire (Q-Les-Q): 93-item self-report instrument, measuring the amount of satisfaction the patient enjoys in different areas of life. Reliable measure for assessing aspects of mental health not covered by other inventories

This study measured the presence and degree of war trauma–related symptoms among Iraq and Afghanistan veterans. The majority of participants experienced a 50% drop in PTSD symptoms by the fourth week, and greater improvements by two months and three months. This included reductions in symptoms of re-experiencing, hypervigilance, avoidance, memory problems, and emotional numbness. Depression was reduced, and quality of life was increased based on the standard measurements.

Rosenthal J, Grosswald, SJ, Ross R, Rosenthal N. Effects of Transcendental Meditation (TM) in Veterans of Operation Enduring Freedom (OEF) and Operation Iraqi Freedom (OIF) with Posttraumatic Stress Disorder (PTSD): A Pilot Study. *Military Medicine* 2011 (in press)

Effects of Transcendental Meditation in Treatment of Post-Vietnam Adjustment

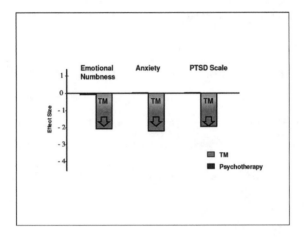

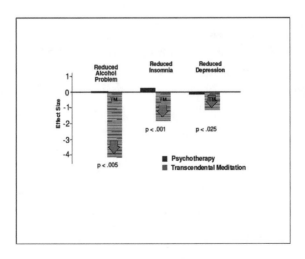

Veterans at a Colorado Vet Center were randomly assigned to either the TM group or a control group receiving standard psychotherapy. After three months, the group practicing the TM technique had significant reductions in PTSD symptoms of emotional numbness, anxiety, startle response, depression, alcohol consumption, and family problems. The TM group also had improvements in sleep and in obtaining/keeping employment. Seventy percent of the TM group reported they no longer needed the services of the Vet Center.

Brooks JS, Scarano T. Transcendental Meditation in the treatment of post-Vietnam adjustment. *Journal of Counseling and Development* 1985 64:212–215

Faster Recovery from a Stressful Stimulus

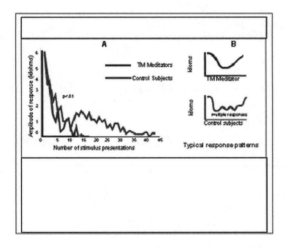

The TM technique results in more rapid recovery from a stressful stimulus, including reversal of symptomatology associated with severe and chronic stress.

Orme-Johnson DW. Autonomic stability and Transcendental Meditation. Psychosomatic Medicine 1973 35(4):341–349

The Transcendental Meditation technique Creates Coherent Functioning of the Brain

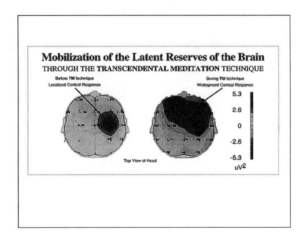

During the practice of the Transcendental Meditation technique there is an increase in the areas of the cortex taking part in perception of specific information, and an increase in functional relationship between the two hemispheres. This creates improved moral reasoning, creativity, and problem solving.

Proceedings of the International Symposium Physiological and Biochemical Basis of Brain Activity, St. Petersburg, Russia (June 22–24, 1992); 2nd Russian-Swedish Symposium New Research in Neurobiology, Moscow, Russia (May 19–21, 1992)

EEG Patterns of Different Meditation Practices

Tibetan Buddhism "unconditional loving kindness and compassion"	Concentration	High 40 Hz EEG activity	Localized attention to detail of experience
Insight, Vipsassana, Mindfulness	Observation	Frontal theta	Attention and emotion centers
Transcendental Meditation	Effortless Transcending	High frontal alpha coherence and higher frontal-posterior phase synchrony	Global coherence

Different meditation techniques have correspondingly different effects on the brain. Techniques of concentration create brain activity corresponding with localized attention. Meditation that involves observation of the body or actions involves primarily the attention and emotion centers of the brain. The Transcendental Meditation technique activates the whole brain, creating total brain coherence.

Comparison of EEG Patterns Among Different Meditation Practices

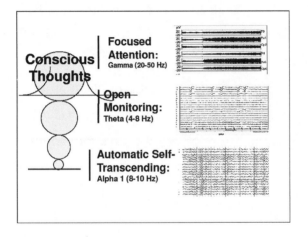

Meditation techniques can be classified into three categories. Techniques that involve Focused Attention are techniques requiring concentration. This form of meditation shows brain activity associated with focused thinking. Meditation types such as mindfulness or Vipassana activate brainwaves associated with drowsiness. The Transcendental Meditation technique is classified as Automatic Self-Transcending, meaning the effect happens effortlessly without controlling the mind. The brain activity associated with TM is synchronistic activation of the whole brain, indicating integrated functioning of the brain.

Travis F, Shear J. Focused attention, open monitoring and automatic self-transcending: Categories to organize meditations from Vedic, Buddhist and Chinese traditions. *Consciousness and Cognition* 2010

Increased Frontal Brain Coherence

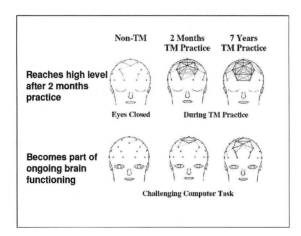

Increase frontal coherence is seen within two months' practice of the Transcendental Meditation technique. The coherent pattern of functioning continues to develop and become part of ongoing brain functioning during activity.

Travis FT, Arenander A. Cross-sectional and longitudinal study of effects of Transcendental Meditation practice on interhemispheric frontal asymmetry and frontal coherence. *International Journal of Neuroscience* 2006 116(12):1519–1538

Effectiveness in Reducing Trait Anxiety: Meta-Analysis

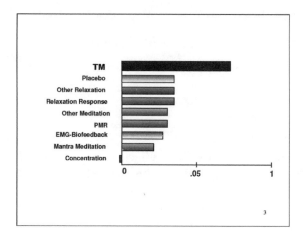

This meta-analysis analyzed virtually all of the published studies at the time that met basic design criteria.   TM showed approximately two times greater response in reducing anxiety (twice the effect size) compared to other techniques.   The study controlled for experimental design and various other potential confounders.

Orme-Johnson, DW.   Medical care utilization and the Transcendental Meditation program.   *Psychosomatic Medicine* 1987 49(1):493–507

Reduced Response to Pain

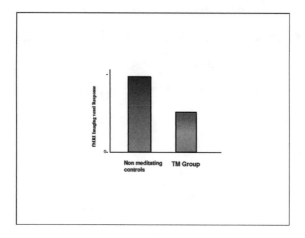

The Transcendental Meditation technique showed 40 to 50 percent fewer voxels responding to pain in the thalamus and total brain than in healthy matched controls. The Transcendental Meditation program appears to longitudinally reduce the brain's response to acute pain along major sectors of the affective dimension of the pain matrix.

Johnson DW, Schneider RH, Son YD, Nidich S, Cho Z. Neuroimaging of meditation's effect on brain reactivity to pain. *Cognitive Neuroscience and Neuropsychology* 2006 17:1359–1363

Meta-Analysis of Reduced Alcohol Abuse

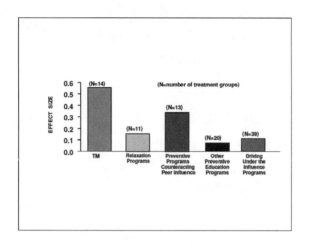

This meta-analysis of 24 studies compared the effectiveness of different approaches for reducing alcohol and illegal drug use. These findings not only show large reductions in the use of alcohol and other non-prescribed drugs with the practice of the TM technique but also show the TM technique to be significantly more effective than the other approaches.

Alexander CN, Robinson P, Rainforth MV. Treating and preventing alcohol, nicotine, and drug abuse through Transcendental Meditation: a review and statistical meta-analysis. *Alcoholism Treatment Quarterly* 1994 11(1/2):13–87

Decreased Health Care Utilization in all Categories

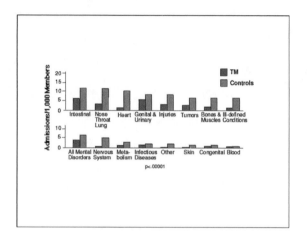

Using Blue Cross Blue Shield data, 2,000 individuals practicing Transcendental Meditation were matched with controls for age, demographic status, occupation, and health insurance characteristics. Over a 5-year period, Transcendental Meditation meditators consistently had less than half as many hospitalizations as the other groups.

Orme-Johnson DW.   Medical care utilization and the Transcendental Meditation program.   *Psychosomatic Medicine* 1987 49(1):493–507

References

Anderson JW, Liu C, Kryscio RJ. Blood pressure response to Transcendental Meditation: A meta-analysis. *American Journal of Hypertension* 2008 21:310–316

Alexander CN, Robinson P, Rainforth MV. Treating and preventing alcohol, nicotine, and drug abuse through Transcendental Meditation: a review and statistical meta-analysis. *Alcoholism Treatment Quarterly* 1994 11(1/2):13–87

Barnes VA, Treiber FA, Kapuku G. Impact of Transcendental Meditation on left ventricular mass in African American adolescents. *Annals of Behavioral Medicine* 2009 37(Supplement):S195

Barnes VA, Schneider RH, Alexander CN, Rainforth M, Staggers F, Salerno J. Impact of Transcendental Meditation on mortality in older African Americans with hypertension— eight-year follow-up. *Journal of Social Behavior and Personality* 2005 17(1):201–216

Brooks JS, Scarano T. Transcendental Meditation in the treatment of post-Vietnam adjustment. *Journal of Counseling and Development* 1985 64:212–215

Castillo-Richmond A, Schneider RH, Alexander CN, Cook R, Myers H, Nidich S, *et al.* Effects of stress reduction on carotid atherosclerosis in hypertensive African Americans. *Stroke* 2000 31(3):568–573

Travis FT, Wallace RK. Autonomic and EEG patterns during eyes-closed rest and Transcendental Meditation (TM) practice: a basis for a neural model of TM practice. *Consciousness and Cognition* 1999 8(3):302–318

Eppley K, Abrams A, Shear J. Differential effects of relaxation techniques on trait anxiety: a meta-analysis. *Journal of Clinical Psychology* 1989 45(6):957–974

Herron RE, Hillis SL, Mandarino JV, Orme-Johnson DW, Walton KG. The impact of the Transcendental Meditation program on government payments to physicians in Quebec. *American Journal of Health Promotion* 1996 10(3):208–216

Herron RE, Hillis SL. The impact of the Transcendental Meditation program on government payments to physicians in Quebec: an update—accumulative decline of 55% over a 6-year period. *American Journal of Health Promotion* 2000 14(5):284–291

Jevning R, Anand R, Beidebach M, Fernando G. Effects on regional cerebral blood flow of Transcendental Meditation. *Physiology and Behavior* 1996 59(3):399–402

Jevning R, Pirkle H, Wilson AF. Behavioural alteration of plasma phenylalanine concentration. *Physiology and Behavior* 1977 19(5):611–614

Jevning R, Wallace RK, Beidebach M. The physiology of meditation: a review. A wakeful hypometabolic integrated response. *Neuroscience and Biobehavioral Reviews* 1992 16(3):415–424

Jevning R, Wells I, Wilson AF, Guich S. Plasma thyroid hormones, thyroid stimulating hormone, and insulin during acute hypometabolic state in man. *Physiology and Behavior* 1987 40(5):603–606

Jevning R, Wilson AF, Davidson JM. Adrenocortical activity during meditation. *Hormones and Behavior* 1978 10(1):54–60

Mulhall, E. Women Warriors. Iraq and Afghanistan Veterans of America Issue Report, Oct. 2009

Orme-Johnson DW, Walton KG. All approaches to preventing and reversing the effects of stress are not the same. *American Journal of Health Promotion* 1998 12(5):297–299

Orme-Johnson DW. Autonomic stability and Transcendental Meditation. *Psychosomatic Medicine* 1973 35(4):341–349

Orme-Johnson DW. Medical care utilization and the Transcendental Meditation program. *Psychosomatic Medicine* 1987 49(1):493–507

Rosenthal J, Grosswald, SJ, Ross R, Rosenthal N. Effects of Transcendental Meditation (TM) in Veterans of Operation Enduring Freedom (OEF) and Operation Iraqi Freedom (OIF) with Posttraumatic Stress Disorder (PTSD): A Pilot Study, 2010 (in press)

Roth, R. *Maharishi Mahesh Yogi's TM Transcendental Meditation*. Fairfield, IA: MUM Press, 2006

Stiglitz JE, Bilmes LL. *The Three Trillion Dollar War*. New York: W.W. Norton & Company, 2008

Travis FT. From I to I: concepts of Self on an object-referral/ self-referral continuum. In AP Prescott (ed.), *The Concept of Self in Psychology*. New York: Nova Publishing, 2006

Travis FT. Relationship between meditation practice and transcendent states of consciousness. *Biofeedback* 2009 (in press)

Travis FT, Arenander A. Cross-sectional and longitudinal study of effects of Transcendental Meditation practice on inter-hemispheric frontal asymmetry and frontal coherence. *International Journal of Neuroscience* 2006 116(12):1519–1538

Travis F, Harung H, Blank W. Higher development and leadership: toward brain measures of managerial capacity. *Journal of Business and Psychology* 2009 (in press)

Travis FT, Arenander A, DuBois D. Psychological and physiological characteristics of a proposed Object-Referral/Self-Referral continuum of self-awareness. *Consciousness and Cognition* 2004 13(2):401–420

Travis FT, Arenander A. Cross-sectional and longitudinal study of effects of Transcendental Meditation practice on inter-hemispheric frontal asymmetry and frontal coherence. *International Journal of Neuroscience* 2006 116(12):1519–1538

Travis FT, Haaga DH, Hagelin JS, Tanner M, Arenander A, Nidich S, *et al.* A self-referential default brain state: patterns of coherence, power, and eLORETA sources during eyes-closed rest and the Transcendental Meditation practice. *Cognitive Processes* 2009 (in press)

Dillbeck MC, Orme-Johnson DW. Physiological differences between Transcendental Meditation and rest. *American Psychologist* 1987 42(9):879–881

Travis F, Haaga DA, Hagelin JS, Tanner M, Nidich S, Gaylord-King C, *et al.* Effects of Transcendental Meditation practice on brain functioning and stress reactivity in college students. *International Journal of Psychophysiology* 2009 (in press)

Zoroya, G. Thousands strain Fort Hood's mental health system. USA Today. Aug. 23, 2010
http://www.usatoday.com/news/military/2010-08-23-1Aforthood23_CV_N.htm

For more information

email
Info@operationwarriorwellness.org

or visit
www.operationwarriorwellness.org